I0416449

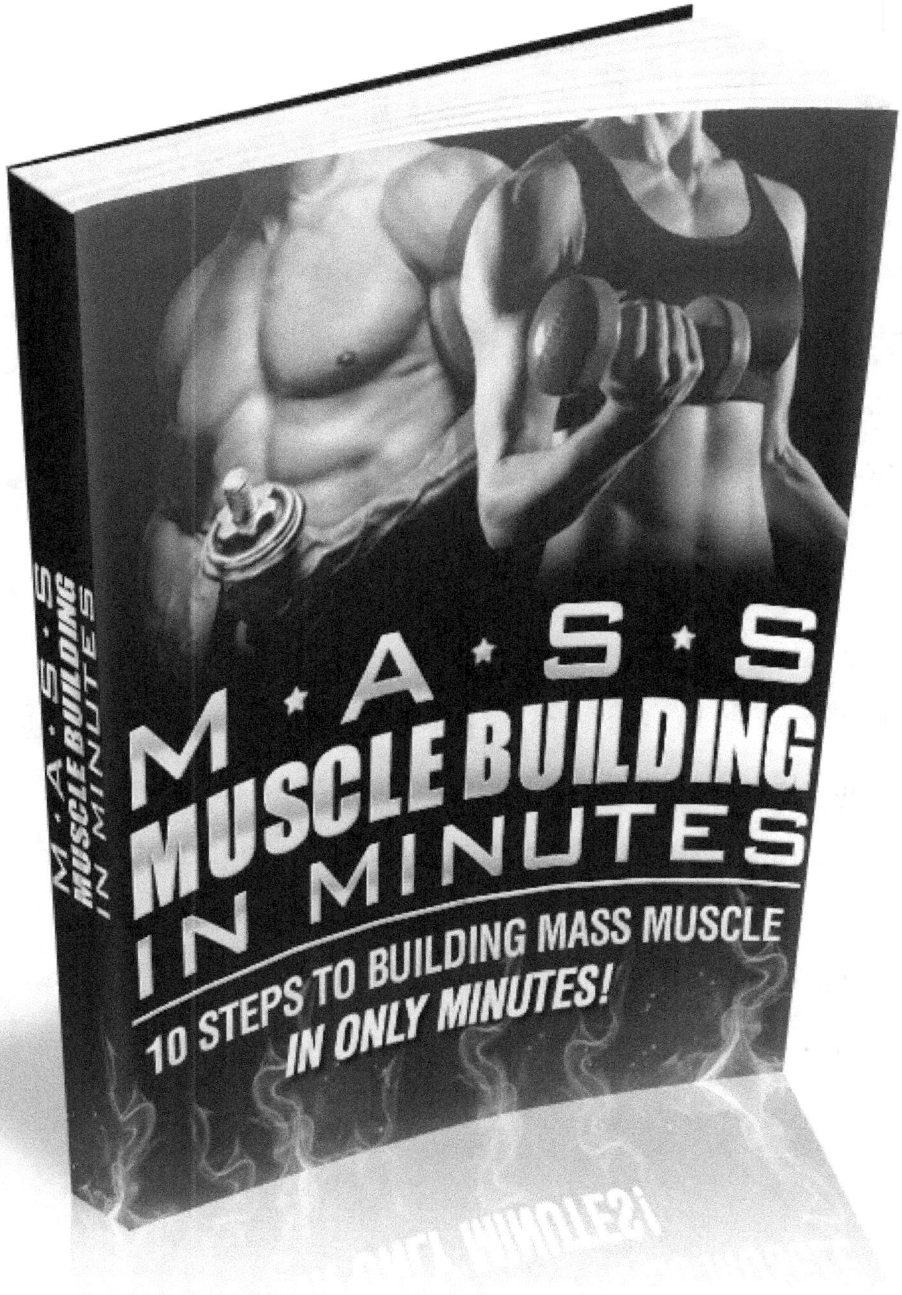

M·A·S·S
MUSCLE BUILDING
IN MINUTES

10 STEPS TO BUILDING MASS MUSCLE
IN ONLY MINUTES!

Copyright © 2013

All rights reserved. No part of this book may be reproduced, stored in a retrieval system, or transmitted in any form or by any means, electronic, mechanical, photocopying, recording, scanning, or otherwise, without the prior written permission of the publisher.

Disclaimer

All the material contained in this book is provided for educational and informational purposes only. No responsibility can be taken for any results or outcomes resulting from the use of this material. While every attempt has been made to provide information that is both accurate and effective, the author does not assume any responsibility for the accuracy or use/misuse of this information.

Table of Contents

INTRODUCTION

Six day a week gym sessions lifting weights lasting nearly two hours followed by marathon cardio. Complicated split training programs, twice a day training, Olympic lifts, German Volume Training. I've had the pleasure (and sometimes the misfortune) of trying them all in my quest for the perfect workout plan.

What if I told you against tradition and what may seem like common sense, that the best way to get big fast is to actually train much, much less, but with total effort and focus?

That this method has been developed and followed since the late 1960's, is more akin to a science than an art form and some of the top bodybuilders of all time have been its advocates?

That the results when followed heroically are mind blowing?

It's all true. Welcome to Mass Muscle Building In Minutes.

By the time you're done you'll be able to use these principles to quickly get huge - all while spending a ridiculously short amount of time in the gym.

If you have what it takes to put in the hardcore work HIT demands that is!

Into High Intensity Training

HIT was first introduced to the bodybuilding and fitness world in 1971 by genius super eccentric training guru Art Jones. Jones was a real maverick. The brains behind the first brand of weight lifting machines that weren't garbage, Nautilus (his son also developed Hammer Strength), Jones was a man possessed with the idea of finding the perfect training program.

Armed with desire, a formidable I.Q. and a near limitless bank account to fund studies and pay athletes Jones eventually came up with the HIT principles. To say these were groundbreaking in those early days of bodybuilding is very much an understatement!

Later on HIT was really expanded and perfected by

Jones's star pupil one of the best bodybuilders who has ever lived Mike Mentzer. Mike was as intelligent and opinionated as he was talented and dedicated. I'd suggest taking a good look at Mike in his prime if you have any doubts what this sort of training is capable of.

Make sure you check out Dorian Yates, Casey Viator and the immortal Clarence Bass too.

Oh, before I forget are you curious what gave Jones his initial inspiration to move in the direction of HIT? Watching his PET gorilla (who weighed over 200kgs) doing one armed pull ups for fun. Jones figured if his gorilla didn't need high rep workouts to be massively powerful, why should anyone else! I told you he was eccentric, didn't I?

What Makes HIT - HIT!

Here's the foundation of High Intensity Training in a nutshell. We'll give more details as we go deeper into our Guide...

* Training Must Be Intense. For this type of training to work its magic, training must be as intense as possible.

This means total exertion until you absolutely can't do any more work. Training to failure is the rule with HIT, not the exception!

* Training Sessions Must Be Short. Training as intensely as HIT demands makes it necessary that your training sessions are short. If you can spend an hour or two in the gym you are not coming close to training intensely enough for HIT. Your workouts need to be short and severe.

* Training Must Be Infrequent. It pays to think of HIT being an equal mix of intensity and recovery. When you are training HIT style you need to train much less to allow your body to recover and grow to its potential. This means only a few sessions a week, unlike traditional bodybuilding methods which almost always end up in the dreaded "over training" zone.

Ready to get Intense with HIT? Good so am I! Read on...

CHAPTER 1 – LESS IS MORE? THE SCIENCE OF HIT

When you first come across the idea of "less, but intense is more" training you can hardly be blamed if you have some initial skepticism. I know I did, after being nearly raised on a diet of bodybuilding magazines that generally pushed ideas that were nearly exactly opposite to HIT.

Seeing is believing, but it's good to know that there is science that backs up the results we see from this training in the gym. Let's take a look. Afterward we'll browse some of the many benefits of this training lifestyle!

HIT is the Science of Bodybuilding

* The Science Behind Intensity. HIT advocates define intensity as training to failure, which is a definition that's not always accepted and used by science and strength training journals. Frankly, our HIT definition makes much more sense than the various ones used by these egg head types. Training to failure as a means towards

building muscle mass quickly has been studied in a series of Journal of Strength and Conditioning Research articles by JM Willardson.

Willardson found himself surprised to end up in agreement with the HIT training theories of Jones and Metzner when he saw a 9.5% increase in power compared to a 5% increase in the same time period by those following more traditional training programs! This backs up exactly what we've seen in the gym! And in the mirror.

* The Science Behind Low Volume. The HIT idea of very low sets for each exercise is an area that is most often attacked by HIT's critics. It's also an area that has returned some of the most promising scientific studies. The Journal of Sports Medicine and the Journal of Exercise Physiology, which are two of the highest regarded journals in the sports and fitness fields both have turned out articles supporting HIT's very low set protocol as being optimal for athletic development!

* The Science Behind Rest. Extended rest days between training sessions has been a key principle we've seen behind the success of HIT over the years. The Journal of

Sports Medicine has featured a series of acclaimed articles by M.J. Cleak that laid out in great detail the fact that when muscles are rested 96 hours between sessions they make strength progressions at a much quicker pace. This is HIT theory confirmed.

Find this intriguing? Mike Mentzer famously wrote a book titled "Science of Bodybuilding" which I'd highly suggest for further HIT reading after our Guide here, of course. It expertly breaks down the science behind HIT principles in great detail. Check it out!

Benefits of HIT

Now that we've seen the science behind high intensity training, let's finish up this chapter with some of the proven benefits of HIT. We enjoy them and you can too!

* Workout Times are Slashed. You spend much less time in the gym training HIT style. A few hours a week as compared to what seems like a part time job with other bodybuilding training methods. This gives us lots more time to devote to other important things, to relax or even to have fun!

* Over training is Never an Issue. Nothing will stunt your muscle growth, strength gains or injure you quicker than over training! With high intensity training you will almost never over train when the principles are followed correctly.

* Joints Stay Protected. Many joint (knee, elbow, shoulder) injuries are from high rep grinding over the years. With HIT training your joints don't receive this type of grinding day in and out. This equals less injuries.

* You Grow and become more Powerful Quickly. This is the primary reason most of us follow HIT. Try HIT and you will become a believer!

Science and real world results. It doesn't get much better.

CHAPTER 2 –DEBUNKING MYTHS OF THE MARATHON WORKOUT

It's safe to say you shouldn't believe about 75% of the things you read in the magazines, books and especially the websites put out by the followers of marathon workout ideas. They don't work and they may get you hurt.

Put on your seat belt while we debunk four of their favorite body building myths!

1. You Need a PUMP to Gain Muscle. If I had a dollar every time I heard a very skinny weightlifter doing 15 rep sets of bicep curls say this, I'd be opening a chain of hardcore gyms very shortly. This myth goes all the way back to Arnold and Pumping Iron. One Arnold didn't mention, which he later admitted, is that he was using large amounts of anabolic steroids while following his "get the pump" work outs that led to his Mr. Olympia winning condition.

The truth is with body building drugs you will likely not over train and any ridiculous work out is much more likely to produce results. Take away the drugs and the "pump" is shown to have no lasting benefit in your quest to get huge. Train for the pump and you will likely stay small forever.

2. High Reps Cut Fat and Give Definition. Ummm.... NO. Having well defined muscle that's visible to the eye is almost completely a matter of how much body fat you are carrying on your frame. Less fat equals more definition. The way to burn fat has zero to do with high rep weight training work outs. You burn fat in three ways: diet, cardio and aggressive supplementation. Anyone who tells you differently is very, very wrong and leading you down the wrong track too!

3. Free Weights are Better Than Machines for Building Muscle. This is a myth most often promoted by the Cross Fit / functional fitness crowd. Remember we are talking about building muscle here - not sport's specific athletic ability. The truth is it all depends on the type of machines available to you as well as how intensely you train on the machine. Mike Mentzer and Dorian Yates became

absolutely huge and won the top body building contests of their time using work outs that consisted of over 75% machine work on Nautilus and Hammer Strength machines respectively. While free weights recruit stabilising muscles, if you generate enough force in the proper movement within a machine, you will be recruiting more muscle fibres. I've gotten in top shape doing the same. Once again how you use the tool is the key - whether free weights or machines, not the tool itself!

4. Marathon Style Weight Training is Safer than HIT Training. The more intense you train the more dangerous correct? No. One or two fully intense sets with total focus on a machine or with a competent spotter is much safer than mindless endless reps and sets done with no focus. Check for yourself the next time you hear someone talk about their gym injury. I bet when you ask what style they were training in it wasn't HIT. In five years of marathon style training I had a dozen injuries... in five years of HIT training none. No style of body building is 100% safe, but HIT is as safe as can be considering. Certainly much safer than what the "go for the pump" crowd are hurting themselves doing every day that's for sure!

Now you have the answers to many of the myths you'll likely hear tossed around the gym about HIT. Knowledge is power!

CHAPTER 3 - THE MOST IMPORTANT THING IN TRAINING...THE MIND!

When it comes to high intensity training it's safe to say - with no mind there's no muscle! The most important thing in HIT is your mind bar none. How best to keep your wits about you and engaged in building the body of your dreams? Read on and find out the top methods I've learned the hard way. Don't be scared to take some notes and bring them with you to your training sessions, they can make all the difference in the world!

* Clarify Your Motivation. Ask yourself and become completely clear on why you are training. The driving force that's going to carry you to the gym when all else fails. This is similar to goal setting in a way, which we'll also in a coming chapter, but much more broad and general. Once you are clear on your motivation take a few minutes to affirm it every day out loud. You can phrase it something like this: "I'm training to get in the

best shape of my life, to be stronger and more attractive." Don't just copy this - your motivation is your own, not mine or anyone else's.

* Make a Training Plan and Stick to It. Human beings despite what your local anarchist may preach instinctively love order. Writing down a training plan and following it is an absolute must for HIT. The more detailed the better. If you've ever seen one of Mentzer's training journals they could double as a book. This keeps your conscious and subconscious mind engaged in your training and paves the way to success.

* Become Accountable. Do you know why more people who work out with personal trainers meet their goals than those without? Not because, in most cases, their trainers have any special knowledge or secrets to share. It's because these people have made themselves accountable to someone to train hard and achieve their goals. This doesn't mean you need to hire a trainer, but it does mean you should grab two people and let them know your training goals and ask them to help keep you accountable towards them. Pick friends or family that will take this responsibility as seriously as you do your training!

* Use Positive Self Talk in the Gym. Do everything you can to silence internal negative dialogue in the gym. The best way sports psychologists have found to do this is through positive self talk while working out. The more martial, aggressive and over the top the better. Think the classic movie Brave Heart my friend. HIT is heroic so think and speak like a hero!

* Model HIT Body Builders who Made It. Read and study high intensity trainers who have developed the type of physique you are aspiring towards. They did it and you can too. The more you read about them the more you will be enlisting your subconscious mind onto your side in your gym wars. This really works so please don't neglect it.

* Enjoy Your Training. Yes our training is intense, but it's also meant to be fun. Do your best to enjoy the gym and not dread it. This will go a very long way towards your building a huge, mighty new self. Loving challenges, and HIT are certainly challenging, it is a trait that will even help you succeed in all other areas of your life once you develop it. How cool is that?

Do you get the idea? Your mind is your most important body part to train! It's also the only body part you should be training seven days a week. Don't neglect it and it won't neglect you.

CHAPTER 4 – RECOVERY! HOW IMPORTANT IS IT? SLEEP AND DAYS OFF BETWEEN WORKOUTS

If intensity is fifty percent of your ultimate HIT results, the other fifty percent is rest and recovery. Some HIT theorists have the balance weighted even further in the direction of rest and recovery to the tune of 75 / 25. No matter how you slice the bread a proper attention to rest and recovery is absolutely vital to your bodybuilding success.

The Importance of Rest Days

HIT philosophy and broader training science both share the opinion you need in the neighborhood of 72 hours of rest between training sessions for each of your body parts for them to be fully recovered. Depending on your own genetics, age and diet you could need even more than this.

Does this mean if you train more often that you won't see results? No, of course not.

What it does mean is that you won't be able to train with maximum intensity if you skip rest days. This is impossible to do because you aren't fully recovered. On top of this you will also not be training in an optimal training environment - where your body grows with the least amount of effort. This is something most of us aspire towards with HIT training. Getting the best results out of the shortest amount of time spent in the gym! After years, it's liberating not spending twenty hours a week at the gym - while getting even better results - believe me!

Sleep and Build Muscle

Even among HIT enthusiasts sometimes the effort to get enough quality sleep is brushed aside and neglected. When you pay attention to your recovery days and combine that with making the most of your sleep you have created the perfect environment to build muscle, so don't make that mistake.

These tips could help!

* Get in at Least Eight Hours of Sleep. Eight hours of solid sleep is really the minimum you need when training heavy and intense. If your lifestyle permits, the closer you can get to ten hours of sleep after hardcore work outs the better. Consider sleeping a second body building session if you must because you won't achieve your goals without it!

* Try to Sleep without Interruption. Broken sleep is not ideal. Turn off the television and let friends and family know you are in training and to only wake you in an emergency. It may take a reminder or two, but eventually they'll get used to your more disciplined sleep schedule.

* Consider Sleep Aide Supplements. If you really need help getting in your rest don't fall into the trap of taking potentially dangerous prescription drugs. These can be addictive and can even cause you to pack on body fat! A better solution? Melatonin, kava kava and Valerian root all can all work wonders towards fighting insomnia. It's a bit beyond the scope of our Guide to dig into specific issues, but they are generally safe and inexpensive. If you need to, do your research and consider adding one (or all) to your own diet program.

It takes a bit of self-discipline to master the winning art of total intensity when training and total relaxation when recovering. With a little practice I have no doubt you can do it. Big rewards await!

CHAPTER 5 – HIT WORKOUTS PART 1

Now we're getting somewhere - our HIT Workouts! In the next two chapters of our guide I'll be breaking down our own version of the high intensity training plan taking the best of old school and new school HIT ideas on the subject. This plan has been proven to be consistently effective for new trainers and old male and female alike.

HIT Workout Part 1 Monday

Unless otherwise noted it should take you roughly four seconds to raise and four seconds to lower your weight in good form. If you are able to complete all the required reps take note in your training journal (you do have a training journal don't you?) and be sure to raise the weight next session.

Intensity! Intensity! Intensity!

1. Leg Extension. Sit at leg extension machine making sure it is adjusted correctly for your height. Jumping on the machine and assuming it's set properly will not allow

you to use the right resistance and will greatly increase your chance of injury. Don't lock your knees as you extend your legs which puts unnecessary stress on your knee joints. Do one set of six to eight reps.

Immediately follow your set with...

2. Leg Presses. This is your primary mass builder for your legs be sure to go as heavy as you are safely able. Come down in a full range of motion - knees to chest. Do one set of six to eight reps.

No rest. Finish your legs with...

3. Calf Raises. Choose the calf raise machine you are most comfortable with. Do one set of eight to ten reps also with a full range of motion.

Rest two to three minutes.

4. Dumbbell Flyes or if available Pec Deck. Fewer gyms seem to have "classic" pec decks available where your arms are in a L shape while squeezing your chest. If you are lucky enough to have a classic pec deck be sure to use it, however I do stress the importance of safe form

with this exercise as it can lead to injury if not performed properly. If not dumbbell flyes also get the job done. Do one set of eight to ten reps.

Immediately follow with...

5. Incline Presses. You can choose dumbbells, barbell or machine incline presses. Be sure to go heavy for a full range of motion. This is one of your best upper body builders so focus on intensity more than ever! Do one set of six to eight reps.

Without rest go to...

6. Body Weight Dips. This is a neglected old school exercise that should be much more popular than it is. Two sets of full range of six to eight reps. When these become too light hang weights from a belt and chain.

Rest two minutes and move on to...

7. Tricep Push downs. Use a standing tricep pushdown machine with a "V" shaped handle. Be sure not to lock your arms at the bottom of each rep - in a few years your elbows will thank you! One set of six to eight reps.

Immediately move on to...

8. Lying Tricep Extensions. Some people choose to call these "skull crushers", but I prefer not to chance fate. Using a barbell bang out one set of six to eight reps again with maximum intensity! Do these loyally and expect horse shoes to be bursting out of your t-shirt sometime soon.

Now go get some rest! Thursday is coming fast.

Is it hard for you to believe half our work out week is already behind us? Well reading about a full force HIT work out and thinking the week is easy and DOING it at maximum intensity are very much different things!

If you are training the way you should be - as well as getting the proper amount of rest - you should start feeling 100% around Wednesday and stronger than ever on Thursday. Which brings us to our next (and final) HIT work out of the week.

Focused and ready? I hope so!

HIT Workout Part 2 (Thursday)

1. Yates Style Barbell or Machine Rows. Rows are to your back what presses are to your chest. We will be performing in the style of former Mr. Olympia and HIT guru Dorian Yates. Take a look at Dorian's back he built doing this version of rows and any doubt you have about your hand position will vanish. How do we do Yates rows?

Simple. With your palms facing up - the opposite direction most people have their palms facing while doing this popular exercise. Dorian credits this variant for not only giving him perhaps the best back in body building history, but also for being his primary bicep mass builder. Do two full range of motion sets of six to eight heavy reps each. Don't neglect your intensity!

Without rest move to...

2. Lat Pull Downs. Be sure the seat is set to the correct position for your height. Pull down to the top of your chest - NOT behind your neck. More injuries have occurred from behind the neck pull downs than any other exercise. Do two sets of six to eight reps.

Immediately perform...

3. Dead lifts. Keep your knees bent. If you have any history of lower back pain wear a weight lifting belt. Do two sets of eight to ten reps. This is an exercise when done with focus will build full body power. If you aspire to be powerful don't neglect your dead lifts!

Rest two to three minutes and move on to...

4. Machine or Barbell Shrugs. Use wrist wraps if you need them to shrug maximum weight. Full range of motion with a one second pause on top. Two sets of six to eight reps. Nothing radiates HIT like well developed traps which is what these will give you, fast!

Go right to...

5. Dumbbell Shoulder Press. Feel free to substitute machine shoulder presses if like many of us you have rotator cuff problems. Stop when your elbows are in a straight line with your upper chest, falling below is inviting injury. One set of six to eight reps.

Rest two to three minutes. Move on to...

6. Barbell Curls. Please don't cheat by swinging your back - use a heavy weight, but one you are curling with your biceps NOT your entire body's momentum! Also be sure to use a full range of motion. This is a exercise where many men let ego rather than true strength dictate the weight they use. Don't be one of them. Two sets of six to eight reps.

Rest one minute, then finish your work out with...

7. Crunches. Three sets to failure of lying floor crunches for your abdominals. Avoid ab machines which are generally pretty useless!

That's it your HIT week is done. I'm dying to know how you feel after your first week of high intensity training insanity!

CHAPTER 7 – EAT TO GROW - HIGH CALORIE, MASS DIET

I have some bad news for some of us. Muscle doesn't come from the void and just appear on our bodies out of nowhere! Even with our following all the HIT principles in our guide so far we are not going to get huge quickly if we're eating like rabbits. Calories, protein and frequent meals are the building blocks that our high intensity training and dedicated rest and recovery will carve a Herculean physique out of.

Keep these broad based mass building diet tips in mind and expect to have to buy a new larger wardrobe fast!

* Raise Your Calories. Okay, first the obvious. When looking to put on mass, you need to boost your calorie intake. My suggestion is to start with an even 1000 extra calories a day. Does this sound like a lot? Well it may, but it works. In fact if you see your weight rising without putting on an excessive amount of body fat tag on another 500 calories a day the following week. Some of us can even go an extra 500 calories beyond this point.

Genetics and our eating habits all play a role here, so individual needs vary greatly in this area.

* Eat Frequently. Splitting your calories up over six evenly spaced meals (while you are awake at least) provides the best meal schedule for mass building. Your body is kept constantly fed which boosts recovery. A welcome side effect in this eating schedule is that it actually works against fat building as long as your diet is relatively clean. Junk food makes you fat - not eating more frequently.

* Protein is King. Your primary muscle builder is protein. A good target is 1.5 to 2 grams of protein per pound you weigh. Divide this between all six meals. Food protein is best, but a shake or two a day won't hurt and is certainly preferable than missing your target amount. When in doubt eat (or drink) more protein!

* Consider Creatine. I've purposely avoided the minefield that is today's supplement industry, but there are two supplements for mass gain nearly every expert agrees works and works well. The first is creatine monohydrate. For about 85% of us (the other 15% can't digest it properly) creatine will help us build quick muscle and

speed recovery. Take five grams a day with grape juice and food for best results.

* Add Fish Oil When Bulking. My final supplement suggestion - add three to five grams of fish oil to your diet every day. Recent studies have shown a solid dose of fish oil not only works near miracles for reducing the amount of time you need to rest between training sessions, but also tremendously boosts a man's hormonal levels on par with some formerly legal pro-hormones and testosterone boosters. Fish oil is much safer than any of those types of things as well!

* Final Tip: Eat (Relatively) Clean. A mass building phase is not the time to be cutting out all carbs or following excessively strict diet protocols beyond those you have already read here, but it isn't the time to overdose on fast food either. Eat clean six days a week focusing on lean proteins and moderate carbs and fats. Pick one day as your cheat day and eat as you please, within reason.

HIT means short and infrequent gym sessions. It doesn't mean you can ignore basic mass building diet discipline. Stay focused, pay attention to what's on your plate and watch yourself grow big time.

CHAPTER 8 - TO DO CARDIO OR NOT TO DO CARDIO?

Cardio and high intensity training. Believe it or not a somewhat controversial subject in HIT circles through the years. Both Art Jones and Mike Mentzer have spoken for and against it at various times. Current experts on HIT have given radically different views on the subject as well. So what follows is both a middle of the road approach to cardio as well as my own opinion based on personal experience and the experience of the many people I've trained with great results.

Ideas on Cardio and HIT

* Pass on the Cardio if Already Lean. First things first. We are not endurance athletes we are body builders, for the most part, striving to put on quality lean muscle. What this means is that we need to focus on our primary goal of mass building and reject the ridiculous habits of mainstream body builders (most of whom only get truly big while on anabolics or if they possess seriously good genetic gifts!). One of these foolish habits is doing cardio

while already lean and trying to bulk up. Not even professional body builders attempt to do this. I've found ten percent body fat a nice number to avoid any cardio at all while under, if getting bigger is a goal.

* Do the Minimum Amount of Cardio Possible. If we do need to add cardio to our high intensity training sessions we need to do so in a way that doesn't drive us into over training. Six days of hour long step master cardio ala Muscle and Fitness programs will melt away our hard earned muscle. Rest days need to be free of high intensity cardio or else they aren't rest days. Remember adequate recovery is a pillar of getting the most out of HIT.

* Do Your Cardio after your HIT. Higher intensity cardio, should you need or want it, before your HIT sessions is a bad idea that can make your training intensity suffer. Schedule your cardio after HIT or, better yet, follow the low impact "Dorian" / HIT cardio method in our next tip.

* Follow the Example of Dorian Yates. Famously, Dorian Yates packed on a level of muscle unseen in body building in the 1990's following a full on HIT program. He also became lean enough to secure multiple Mr. Olympias. His

cardio solution? Waking up a bit earlier in the morning and taking a brisk low impact walk four days a week before breakfast. When combined with HIT in the gym, a clean diet and fat burning supplementation this was more than enough to get Dorian ripped. Now we probably don't possess Dorian's one in a million genetics, but I've used the same plan and leaned out. So have the majority of my training clientele while following HIT. This is accomplished without losing any of our lean muscle, over training or shackling us to a treadmill at the gym. Try it and see what you think!

Your approach to cardio is an area where your genetics, your body weight and attitudes toward training will play a huge role in what direction you choose to take. None will disqualify you as a HIT enthusiast. Feel free to experiment until you find what works best for you!

CHAPTER 9 - LONG TERM GOAL SETTING AND ACHIEVING RESULTS

Attempting to make dramatic progress with HIT or any other training system is next to impossible until you master the art and science of effective goal setting.

It's the one quality if you do a bit of research you find all the personalities who rose to dominance in bodybuilding share in common. With HIT being even more cerebral than more conventional training methods it's no surprise the high intensity gurus had and practiced the best goal setting ideas and methods. Here's their top ideas on the subject. Follow them closely and your mental game will be backing up your physical game 100%!

* Set Big Goals to Cover Your Big Vision. Your big goals give you a long term target to aim for and can serve as a huge motivational force. Personally I like to set six month, one year and five year fitness and bodybuilding goals. Looking back over the years this has proven to be very successful and most of these long term goals in the past have been met. Dorian Yates was a huge HIT

advocate of this through his entire career and training life. We see how well this practice help Dorian succeed don't we?

* Break Your Big Goals into Monthly and Weekly Goals. Breaking your long term targets into more easily achievable monthly and weekly steps, is a sure way to move progressively forward in a measurable way. You can even set daily fitness and training goals to break the process down even more!

* Frame Your Goals in Positive Language. Sports psychology and mental toughness experts have proven that goals are much more likely to be achieved when they are set in positive language. This means using words like "get stronger" rather than "not be weak" for example. Our minds respond more efficiently to positive language so be sure to use this to your high intensity training advantage.

* Always Put Your Goals on Paper. Pen and paper are your best friends with goal setting. Not only does this keep them fresh in mind as long as you refer back to your notebook periodically, but it's also not a bad idea to make copies of your goals and take them with you both to work

and to the gym. This will do wonders towards keeping you focused!

* Have Quarterly Update Meetings with a Training Mentor. If you have the opportunity to work with a coach, trainer or even a friend who hits the gym with you let them know about the goals you have set and meet with them every few months and discuss how progress is going. In return if it's a friend or family member you can provide the same sounding board about their own training progress. It can't be stressed enough that being held accountable to someone you respect can mean all the difference when going gets tough to help you push through the boundaries and make superhuman changes in your life!

Once you apply these goal setting ideas you will find results coming from your HIT work outs coming quicker than ever. Many of them can be used to make big improvements outside of the gym as well. Try them out and I think you'll be hooked.

CONCLUSION - TRAIN SAFE, TRAIN HARD AND START TODAY

Congratulations, you've made it through Mass Muscle Building In Minutes and learned some of the roughest and toughest bodybuilding methods ever developed. How do you feel? I bet once you put them to good use your physique will never be the same in all the best ways!

Before I leave you to your exciting HIT adventures, I just wanted to bounce three last important HIT rules off of you. Pay close attention, if you apply them right away you're nearly guaranteed long lasting training success. Here they go...

Rule 1: Train Safe. Please repeat after me: "If I foolishly injure myself and can't train, all my hard work could be for nothing!" It's a seriously common problem for ego or machismo to kick in at the gym and the idea of training safely to be totally ignored. Some HIT trainers slide into this trap confusing recklessness for intensity. Don't be one of them. Blowing out a knee, tearing a rotator cuff, straining a lower back and worse are all largely avoidable if you are focused and serious while weight lifting. Make sure you warm up thoroughly, never go too heavy, always use a competent spotter and be sure any machine you use functions properly before you risk your safety training on it. Injuries occur even in the best of circumstances, but as smart athletes it is our job to reduce them to the minimum amount possible.

Rule 2: Train Hard. You are not doing HIT unless you are training as hard as you can imagine. As long as safety is never compromised we need to push the intensity element of our work out sessions to the limit. Once you have mastered the HIT principles in our guide do some exploring in the neighborhood of forced reps, negatives and rest / pauses. All advanced HIT techniques that can explode your training to an even more hard and intense level in the years to come. Think Nietzsche - "That which does not kill me only serves to make me stronger" or the HIT bodybuilder mantra - "Go hard or go home!"

Rule 3: Start Today. In the drive towards anything that really matters in life, including developing the powerful great looking body of your dreams, your number one enemy is procrastination! It's all too easy to say "I'll start tomorrow," "I'll start on Monday" or "I'll start on the first of the month" which just sets you up to postpone pursuing your goals even longer when you put things off again. And again. The only solution is to smash through this tendency towards mediocrity and start today! Not tomorrow, next week or next year. Once the beast of procrastination is slain, literally anything is possible in life once you put your mind to. The formula for success: set smart goals and take immediate action. Judge results and repeat until goal is achieved. Then set targets on new bigger goals!

Are you ready to start living the high intensity training lifestyle? I hope so and I hope you like the awesome HIT tools I provided for you here in our guide. Stay in touch I'd love to hear feedback about how well your training is going!

www.ingramcontent.com/pod-product-compliance
Lightning Source LLC
Chambersburg PA
CBHW082246310526
45795CB00015B/3065